## THIS CAREGIVERS JOURNAL BELONGS TO

_____

_____

_____

## CONTACT DETAILS

_____

_____

_____

_____

# DEDICATION

This Caregiver Log Journal is dedicated to all the caregivers out there who want to track their client's care and document their findings in the process.

You are my inspiration for producing books and I'm honored to be a part of keeping all of your Caregiver notes and records organized.

This journal notebook will help you record your details about tracking your client's daily care.

Thoughtfully put together with these sections to record: Name & Date, Toileting, Meals & Snacks, Activities, Appointments , Health Concerns, Plans For Tomorrow, Supplies Needed Soon, Pain, Alert Levels, and much more!

# HOW TO USE THIS BOOK

The purpose of this book is to keep all of your Caregiving notes all in one place. It will help keep you organized.

This Caregiver Log will allow you to accurately document every detail about your Client's Care. It's a great way to chart your course through tracking your caregiving.

Here are examples of the prompts for you to fill in and write about your experience in this book:

* 1. Name & Date

* 2. Toileting

* 3. Times Up In The Night

* 4. Meals Schedule, Snacks, Drinks

* 5. Activities

* 6. Appointments

* 7. Health Concerns

* 8. Plans For Tomorrow

* 9. Pain Level, Happiness Level, Alertness Level

* 10. Supplies Needed Soon

* 11. Medication Taken

* 12. Notes

# Activity & Caregiving Notes for _____ Date: _____

## TOILETING

| TIME | | | | | | | |
|------|--|--|--|--|--|--|--|
| U | | | | | | | |
| BM | | | | | | | |

### TIMES UP DURING THE NIGHT

_____  _____  _____  _____  _____

### TODAY I HAD A SHOWER/WASHED MY HAIR/SPONGE BATH

| Breakfast | |
|-----------|--|
| AM Snack | |
| Lunch | |
| PM Snack | |
| Dinner | |
| Drinks | |

### ACTIVITIES & OTHER COMMENTS

_____
_____
_____
_____
_____
_____

APPOINTMENTS: _____

HEALTH CONCERNS: _____

PLANS FOR TOMORROW: _____

PAIN LEVEL: _____ HAPPINESS LEVEL: _____ ALERTNESS LEVEL: _____

SUPPLIES NEEDED SOON: _____

MEDICATION TAKEN: _____

### NOTES

_____
_____
_____

# Activity & Caregiving Notes for _____ Date: _____

### TOILETING

| TIME | | | | | | | |
|------|--|--|--|--|--|--|--|
| U | | | | | | | |
| BM | | | | | | | |

### TIMES UP DURING THE NIGHT

_____  _____  _____  _____  _____

### TODAY I HAD A SHOWER/WASHED MY HAIR/SPONGE BATH

| Breakfast | |
|-----------|--|
| AM Snack | |
| Lunch | |
| PM Snack | |
| Dinner | |
| Drinks | |

### ACTIVITIES & OTHER COMMENTS

_____
_____
_____
_____
_____
_____

APPOINTMENTS: _____
HEALTH CONCERNS: _____
PLANS FOR TOMORROW: _____
PAIN LEVEL: _____HAPPINESS LEVEL:_____ALERTNESS LEVEL: _____
SUPPLIES NEEDED SOON: _____
MEDICATION TAKEN: _____

### NOTES

_____
_____
_____

# Activity & Caregiving Notes for _____ Date: _____

## TOILETING

| TIME | | | | | | | |
|------|---|---|---|---|---|---|---|
| U | | | | | | | |
| BM | | | | | | | |

### TIMES UP DURING THE NIGHT

_____  _____  _____  _____  _____

### TODAY I HAD A SHOWER/WASHED MY HAIR/SPONGE BATH

| Breakfast | |
|-----------|---|
| AM Snack | |
| Lunch | |
| PM Snack | |
| Dinner | |
| Drinks | |

### ACTIVITIES & OTHER COMMENTS

_____
_____
_____
_____
_____
_____

APPOINTMENTS: _____
HEALTH CONCERNS: _____
PLANS FOR TOMORROW: _____
PAIN LEVEL: _____HAPPINESS LEVEL:_____ALERTNESS LEVEL: _____
SUPPLIES NEEDED SOON: _____
MEDICATION TAKEN: _____

### NOTES

_____
_____
_____

# Activity & Caregiving Notes for _____ Date: _____

### TOILETING

| TIME | | | | | | | |
|------|--|--|--|--|--|--|--|
| U | | | | | | | |
| BM | | | | | | | |

### TIMES UP DURING THE NIGHT

_____   _____   _____   _____   _____

### TODAY I HAD A SHOWER/WASHED MY HAIR/SPONGE BATH

| Breakfast | |
|-----------|--|
| AM Snack | |
| Lunch | |
| PM Snack | |
| Dinner | |
| Drinks | |

### ACTIVITIES & OTHER COMMENTS

_____
_____
_____
_____
_____
_____

APPOINTMENTS: _____
HEALTH CONCERNS: _____
PLANS FOR TOMORROW: _____
PAIN LEVEL: _____ HAPPINESS LEVEL: _____ ALERTNESS LEVEL: _____
SUPPLIES NEEDED SOON: _____
MEDICATION TAKEN: _____

### NOTES

_____
_____
_____

# Activity & Caregiving Notes for _____ Date: _____

## TOILETING

| TIME | | | | | | | |
|------|--|--|--|--|--|--|--|
| U | | | | | | | |
| BM | | | | | | | |

### TIMES UP DURING THE NIGHT

_____   _____   _____   _____   _____

### TODAY I HAD A SHOWER/WASHED MY HAIR/SPONGE BATH

| Breakfast | |
|-----------|--|
| AM Snack | |
| Lunch | |
| PM Snack | |
| Dinner | |
| Drinks | |

### ACTIVITIES & OTHER COMMENTS

_____

_____

_____

_____

_____

_____

APPOINTMENTS: _____

HEALTH CONCERNS: _____

PLANS FOR TOMORROW: _____

PAIN LEVEL: _____HAPPINESS LEVEL:_____ALERTNESS LEVEL: _____

SUPPLIES NEEDED SOON: _____

MEDICATION TAKEN: _____

### NOTES

_____

_____

_____

# Activity & Caregiving Notes for _____ Date: _____

TOILETING

| TIME | | | | | | | |
|------|--|--|--|--|--|--|--|
| U | | | | | | | |
| BM | | | | | | | |

TIMES UP DURING THE NIGHT

_____   _____   _____   _____   _____

TODAY I HAD A SHOWER/WASHED MY HAIR/SPONGE BATH

| Breakfast | |
|-----------|--|
| AM Snack | |
| Lunch | |
| PM Snack | |
| Dinner | |
| Drinks | |

ACTIVITIES & OTHER COMMENTS

_____

_____

_____

_____

_____

_____

APPOINTMENTS: _____

HEALTH CONCERNS: _____

PLANS FOR TOMORROW: _____

PAIN LEVEL: _____ HAPPINESS LEVEL: _____ ALERTNESS LEVEL: _____

SUPPLIES NEEDED SOON: _____

MEDICATION TAKEN: _____

NOTES

_____

_____

_____

# Activity & Caregiving Notes for _____ Date: _____

### TOILETING

| TIME | | | | | | | |
|------|---|---|---|---|---|---|---|
| U | | | | | | | |
| BM | | | | | | | |

### TIMES UP DURING THE NIGHT

_____    _____    _____    _____    _____

### TODAY I HAD A SHOWER/WASHED MY HAIR/SPONGE BATH

| Breakfast | |
|-----------|---|
| AM Snack | |
| Lunch | |
| PM Snack | |
| Dinner | |
| Drinks | |

### ACTIVITIES & OTHER COMMENTS

_____
_____
_____
_____
_____
_____

APPOINTMENTS: _____

HEALTH CONCERNS: _____

PLANS FOR TOMORROW: _____

PAIN LEVEL: _____ HAPPINESS LEVEL: _____ ALERTNESS LEVEL: _____

SUPPLIES NEEDED SOON: _____

MEDICATION TAKEN: _____

### NOTES

_____
_____
_____

# Activity & Caregiving Notes for _____ Date: _____

## TOILETING

| TIME | | | | | | | |
|---|---|---|---|---|---|---|---|
| U | | | | | | | |
| BM | | | | | | | |

## TIMES UP DURING THE NIGHT

_____   _____   _____   _____   _____

## TODAY I HAD A SHOWER/WASHED MY HAIR/SPONGE BATH

| Breakfast | |
|---|---|
| AM Snack | |
| Lunch | |
| PM Snack | |
| Dinner | |
| Drinks | |

## ACTIVITIES & OTHER COMMENTS

_____
_____
_____
_____
_____
_____

APPOINTMENTS: _____
HEALTH CONCERNS: _____
PLANS FOR TOMORROW: _____
PAIN LEVEL: _____HAPPINESS LEVEL:_____ALERTNESS LEVEL: _____
SUPPLIES NEEDED SOON: _____
MEDICATION TAKEN: _____

## NOTES

_____
_____
_____

# Activity & Caregiving Notes for _____ Date: _____

## TOILETING

| TIME | | | | | | | |
|------|--|--|--|--|--|--|--|
| **U** | | | | | | | |
| **BM** | | | | | | | |

### TIMES UP DURING THE NIGHT

_____  _____  _____  _____  _____

### TODAY I HAD A SHOWER/WASHED MY HAIR/SPONGE BATH

| Breakfast | |
|-----------|--|
| AM Snack | |
| Lunch | |
| PM Snack | |
| Dinner | |
| Drinks | |

### ACTIVITIES & OTHER COMMENTS

_____

_____

_____

_____

_____

_____

APPOINTMENTS: _____

HEALTH CONCERNS: _____

PLANS FOR TOMORROW: _____

PAIN LEVEL: _____ HAPPINESS LEVEL: _____ ALERTNESS LEVEL: _____

SUPPLIES NEEDED SOON: _____

MEDICATION TAKEN: _____

### NOTES

_____

_____

_____

# Activity & Caregiving Notes for _____ Date: _____

## TOILETING

| TIME | | | | | | | | |
|------|--|--|--|--|--|--|--|--|
| U | | | | | | | | |
| BM | | | | | | | | |

### TIMES UP DURING THE NIGHT

_____   _____   _____   _____   _____

### TODAY I HAD A SHOWER/WASHED MY HAIR/SPONGE BATH

| Breakfast | |
|-----------|--|
| AM Snack | |
| Lunch | |
| PM Snack | |
| Dinner | |
| Drinks | |

### ACTIVITIES & OTHER COMMENTS

_____

_____

_____

_____

_____

_____

APPOINTMENTS: _____

HEALTH CONCERNS: _____

PLANS FOR TOMORROW: _____

PAIN LEVEL: _____ HAPPINESS LEVEL: _____ ALERTNESS LEVEL: _____

SUPPLIES NEEDED SOON: _____

MEDICATION TAKEN: _____

### NOTES

_____

_____

_____

# Activity & Caregiving Notes for _____ Date: _____

## TOILETING

| TIME | | | | | | | |
|------|--|--|--|--|--|--|--|
| U | | | | | | | |
| BM | | | | | | | |

TIMES UP DURING THE NIGHT

_____   _____   _____   _____   _____

TODAY I HAD A SHOWER/WASHED MY HAIR/SPONGE BATH

| Breakfast | |
|-----------|--|
| AM Snack | |
| Lunch | |
| PM Snack | |
| Dinner | |
| Drinks | |

## ACTIVITIES & OTHER COMMENTS

_____
_____
_____
_____
_____
_____

APPOINTMENTS: _____
HEALTH CONCERNS: _____
PLANS FOR TOMORROW: _____
PAIN LEVEL: _____HAPPINESS LEVEL:_____ALERTNESS LEVEL: _____
SUPPLIES NEEDED SOON: _____
MEDICATION TAKEN: _____

## NOTES

_____
_____
_____

# Activity & Caregiving Notes for _____ Date: _____

## TOILETING

| TIME | | | | | | |
|------|--|--|--|--|--|--|
| U | | | | | | |
| BM | | | | | | |

### TIMES UP DURING THE NIGHT

_____   _____   _____   _____   _____

### TODAY I HAD A SHOWER/WASHED MY HAIR/SPONGE BATH

| Breakfast | |
|-----------|--|
| AM Snack | |
| Lunch | |
| PM Snack | |
| Dinner | |
| Drinks | |

### ACTIVITIES & OTHER COMMENTS

_____

_____

_____

_____

_____

_____

_____

APPOINTMENTS: _____

HEALTH CONCERNS: _____

PLANS FOR TOMORROW: _____

PAIN LEVEL: _____ HAPPINESS LEVEL: _____ ALERTNESS LEVEL: _____

SUPPLIES NEEDED SOON: _____

MEDICATION TAKEN: _____

### NOTES

_____

_____

_____

# Activity & Caregiving Notes for _____ Date: _____

### TOILETING

| TIME | | | | | | | |
|------|---|---|---|---|---|---|---|
| U | | | | | | | |
| BM | | | | | | | |

### TIMES UP DURING THE NIGHT

_____   _____   _____   _____   _____

### TODAY I HAD A SHOWER/WASHED MY HAIR/SPONGE BATH

| Breakfast | |
|-----------|---|
| AM Snack | |
| Lunch | |
| PM Snack | |
| Dinner | |
| Drinks | |

### ACTIVITIES & OTHER COMMENTS

_____

_____

_____

_____

_____

_____

APPOINTMENTS: _____

HEALTH CONCERNS: _____

PLANS FOR TOMORROW: _____

PAIN LEVEL: _____ HAPPINESS LEVEL: _____ ALERTNESS LEVEL: _____

SUPPLIES NEEDED SOON: _____

MEDICATION TAKEN: _____

### NOTES

_____

_____

_____

# Activity & Caregiving Notes for _____ Date: _____

### TOILETING

| TIME | | | | | | | |
|------|--|--|--|--|--|--|--|
| U | | | | | | | |
| BM | | | | | | | |

### TIMES UP DURING THE NIGHT

_____    _____    _____    _____    _____

### TODAY I HAD A SHOWER/WASHED MY HAIR/SPONGE BATH

| Breakfast | |
|-----------|--|
| AM Snack | |
| Lunch | |
| PM Snack | |
| Dinner | |
| Drinks | |

### ACTIVITIES & OTHER COMMENTS

_____
_____
_____
_____
_____
_____
_____

APPOINTMENTS: _____

HEALTH CONCERNS: _____

PLANS FOR TOMORROW: _____

PAIN LEVEL: _____ HAPPINESS LEVEL: _____ ALERTNESS LEVEL: _____

SUPPLIES NEEDED SOON: _____

MEDICATION TAKEN: _____

### NOTES

_____
_____
_____

# Activity & Caregiving Notes for _____ Date: _____

## TOILETING

| TIME | | | | | | | |
|------|---|---|---|---|---|---|---|
| U | | | | | | | |
| BM | | | | | | | |

### TIMES UP DURING THE NIGHT

_____    _____    _____    _____    _____

### TODAY I HAD A SHOWER/WASHED MY HAIR/SPONGE BATH

| Breakfast | |
|-----------|---|
| AM Snack | |
| Lunch | |
| PM Snack | |
| Dinner | |
| Drinks | |

### ACTIVITIES & OTHER COMMENTS

_____

_____

_____

_____

_____

_____

APPOINTMENTS: _____

HEALTH CONCERNS: _____

PLANS FOR TOMORROW: _____

PAIN LEVEL: _____ HAPPINESS LEVEL: _____ ALERTNESS LEVEL: _____

SUPPLIES NEEDED SOON: _____

MEDICATION TAKEN: _____

### NOTES

_____

_____

_____

# Activity & Caregiving Notes for _____ Date: _____

## TOILETING

| TIME | | | | | | | |
|------|--|--|--|--|--|--|--|
| U | | | | | | | |
| BM | | | | | | | |

### TIMES UP DURING THE NIGHT

_____  _____  _____  _____  _____

### TODAY I HAD A SHOWER/WASHED MY HAIR/SPONGE BATH

| Breakfast | |
|-----------|--|
| AM Snack | |
| Lunch | |
| PM Snack | |
| Dinner | |
| Drinks | |

### ACTIVITIES & OTHER COMMENTS

_____
_____
_____
_____
_____
_____

APPOINTMENTS: _____
HEALTH CONCERNS: _____
PLANS FOR TOMORROW: _____
PAIN LEVEL: _____ HAPPINESS LEVEL: _____ ALERTNESS LEVEL: _____
SUPPLIES NEEDED SOON: _____
MEDICATION TAKEN: _____

### NOTES

_____
_____
_____

# Activity & Caregiving Notes for _____ Date: _____

## TOILETING

| TIME | | | | | | | |
|------|--|--|--|--|--|--|--|
| U | | | | | | | |
| BM | | | | | | | |

### TIMES UP DURING THE NIGHT

_____    _____    _____    _____    _____

### TODAY I HAD A SHOWER/WASHED MY HAIR/SPONGE BATH

| Breakfast | |
|-----------|--|
| AM Snack | |
| Lunch | |
| PM Snack | |
| Dinner | |
| Drinks | |

### ACTIVITIES & OTHER COMMENTS

_____
_____
_____
_____
_____
_____

APPOINTMENTS: _____

HEALTH CONCERNS: _____

PLANS FOR TOMORROW: _____

PAIN LEVEL: _____HAPPINESS LEVEL:_____ALERTNESS LEVEL: _____

SUPPLIES NEEDED SOON: _____

MEDICATION TAKEN: _____

### NOTES

_____
_____
_____

# Activity & Caregiving Notes for _____ Date: _____

### TOILETING

| TIME | | | | | | | |
|------|---|---|---|---|---|---|---|
| U | | | | | | | |
| BM | | | | | | | |

### TIMES UP DURING THE NIGHT

_____   _____   _____   _____   _____

### TODAY I HAD A SHOWER/WASHED MY HAIR/SPONGE BATH

| Breakfast | |
|-----------|---|
| AM Snack | |
| Lunch | |
| PM Snack | |
| Dinner | |
| Drinks | |

### ACTIVITIES & OTHER COMMENTS

_____

_____

_____

_____

_____

_____

APPOINTMENTS: _____

HEALTH CONCERNS: _____

PLANS FOR TOMORROW: _____

PAIN LEVEL: _____ HAPPINESS LEVEL: _____ ALERTNESS LEVEL: _____

SUPPLIES NEEDED SOON: _____

MEDICATION TAKEN: _____

### NOTES

_____

_____

_____

# Activity & Caregiving Notes for _____ Date: _____

## TOILETING

| TIME | | | | | | | |
|------|--|--|--|--|--|--|--|
| U | | | | | | | |
| BM | | | | | | | |

### TIMES UP DURING THE NIGHT

_____  _____  _____  _____  _____

### TODAY I HAD A SHOWER/WASHED MY HAIR/SPONGE BATH

| Breakfast | |
|-----------|--|
| AM Snack | |
| Lunch | |
| PM Snack | |
| Dinner | |
| Drinks | |

### ACTIVITIES & OTHER COMMENTS

_____
_____
_____
_____
_____
_____

APPOINTMENTS: _____
HEALTH CONCERNS: _____
PLANS FOR TOMORROW: _____
PAIN LEVEL: _____ HAPPINESS LEVEL: _____ ALERTNESS LEVEL: _____
SUPPLIES NEEDED SOON: _____
MEDICATION TAKEN: _____

### NOTES

_____
_____
_____

# Activity & Caregiving Notes for _____ Date: _____

## TOILETING

| TIME | | | | | | | |
|------|---|---|---|---|---|---|---|
| U | | | | | | | |
| BM | | | | | | | |

### TIMES UP DURING THE NIGHT

_____    _____    _____    _____    _____

### TODAY I HAD A SHOWER/WASHED MY HAIR/SPONGE BATH

| Breakfast | |
|-----------|---|
| AM Snack | |
| Lunch | |
| PM Snack | |
| Dinner | |
| Drinks | |

### ACTIVITIES & OTHER COMMENTS

_____
_____
_____
_____
_____
_____

APPOINTMENTS: _____
HEALTH CONCERNS: _____
PLANS FOR TOMORROW: _____
PAIN LEVEL: _____HAPPINESS LEVEL:_____ALERTNESS LEVEL: _____
SUPPLIES NEEDED SOON: _____
MEDICATION TAKEN: _____

### NOTES

_____
_____
_____

# Activity & Caregiving Notes for _____ Date: _____

## TOILETING

| TIME | | | | | | | |
|------|--|--|--|--|--|--|--|
| U | | | | | | | |
| BM | | | | | | | |

### TIMES UP DURING THE NIGHT

_____  _____  _____  _____  _____

### TODAY I HAD A SHOWER/WASHED MY HAIR/SPONGE BATH

| Breakfast | |
|-----------|--|
| AM Snack | |
| Lunch | |
| PM Snack | |
| Dinner | |
| Drinks | |

### ACTIVITIES & OTHER COMMENTS

_____

_____

_____

_____

_____

_____

APPOINTMENTS: _____

HEALTH CONCERNS: _____

PLANS FOR TOMORROW:_____

PAIN LEVEL: _____HAPPINESS LEVEL:_____ALERTNESS LEVEL: _____

SUPPLIES NEEDED SOON:_____

MEDICATION TAKEN:_____

### NOTES

_____

_____

_____

# Activity & Caregiving Notes for _____ Date: ____

### TOILETING

| TIME | | | | | | | |
|------|--|--|--|--|--|--|--|
| U | | | | | | | |
| BM | | | | | | | |

### TIMES UP DURING THE NIGHT

_____   _____   _____   _____   _____

### TODAY I HAD A SHOWER/WASHED MY HAIR/SPONGE BATH

| Breakfast | |
|-----------|--|
| AM Snack | |
| Lunch | |
| PM Snack | |
| Dinner | |
| Drinks | |

### ACTIVITIES & OTHER COMMENTS

_____

_____

_____

_____

_____

_____

APPOINTMENTS: _____

HEALTH CONCERNS: _____

PLANS FOR TOMORROW: _____

PAIN LEVEL: _____ HAPPINESS LEVEL: _____ ALERTNESS LEVEL: _____

SUPPLIES NEEDED SOON: _____

MEDICATION TAKEN: _____

### NOTES

_____

_____

_____

# Activity & Caregiving Notes for _____ Date: _____

### TOILETING

| TIME | | | | | | | |
|------|--|--|--|--|--|--|--|
| U | | | | | | | |
| BM | | | | | | | |

### TIMES UP DURING THE NIGHT

_____  _____  _____  _____  _____

### TODAY I HAD A SHOWER/WASHED MY HAIR/SPONGE BATH

| Breakfast | |
|-----------|--|
| AM Snack | |
| Lunch | |
| PM Snack | |
| Dinner | |
| Drinks | |

### ACTIVITIES & OTHER COMMENTS

_____

_____

_____

_____

_____

_____

APPOINTMENTS: _____

HEALTH CONCERNS: _____

PLANS FOR TOMORROW: _____

PAIN LEVEL: _____ HAPPINESS LEVEL:_____ ALERTNESS LEVEL: _____

SUPPLIES NEEDED SOON: _____

MEDICATION TAKEN: _____

### NOTES

_____

_____

_____

# Activity & Caregiving Notes for _____ Date: _____

## TOILETING

| TIME | | | | | | | |
|------|---|---|---|---|---|---|---|
| U | | | | | | | |
| BM | | | | | | | |

### TIMES UP DURING THE NIGHT

_____    _____    _____    _____    _____

### TODAY I HAD A SHOWER/WASHED MY HAIR/SPONGE BATH

| Breakfast | |
|-----------|---|
| AM Snack | |
| Lunch | |
| PM Snack | |
| Dinner | |
| Drinks | |

## ACTIVITIES & OTHER COMMENTS

_____

_____

_____

_____

_____

_____

APPOINTMENTS: _____

HEALTH CONCERNS: _____

PLANS FOR TOMORROW: _____

PAIN LEVEL: _____ HAPPINESS LEVEL: _____ ALERTNESS LEVEL: _____

SUPPLIES NEEDED SOON: _____

MEDICATION TAKEN: _____

## NOTES

_____

_____

_____

# Activity & Caregiving Notes for _____ Date: _____

## TOILETING

| TIME | | | | | | | |
|------|---|---|---|---|---|---|---|
| U | | | | | | | |
| BM | | | | | | | |

### TIMES UP DURING THE NIGHT

_____   _____   _____   _____   _____

### TODAY I HAD A SHOWER/WASHED MY HAIR/SPONGE BATH

| Breakfast | |
|-----------|---|
| AM Snack | |
| Lunch | |
| PM Snack | |
| Dinner | |
| Drinks | |

### ACTIVITIES & OTHER COMMENTS

_____
_____
_____
_____
_____
_____
_____

APPOINTMENTS: _____
HEALTH CONCERNS: _____
PLANS FOR TOMORROW: _____
PAIN LEVEL: _____ HAPPINESS LEVEL: _____ ALERTNESS LEVEL: _____
SUPPLIES NEEDED SOON: _____
MEDICATION TAKEN: _____

### NOTES

_____
_____
_____

# Activity & Caregiving Notes for _____ Date: _____

## TOILETING

| TIME | | | | | | | |
|------|---|---|---|---|---|---|---|
| **U** | | | | | | | |
| **BM** | | | | | | | |

### TIMES UP DURING THE NIGHT

_____    _____    _____    _____    _____

### TODAY I HAD A SHOWER/WASHED MY HAIR/SPONGE BATH

| | |
|---|---|
| **Breakfast** | |
| **AM Snack** | |
| **Lunch** | |
| **PM Snack** | |
| **Dinner** | |
| **Drinks** | |

### ACTIVITIES & OTHER COMMENTS

_____

_____

_____

_____

_____

_____

_____

APPOINTMENTS: _____

HEALTH CONCERNS: _____

PLANS FOR TOMORROW: _____

PAIN LEVEL: _____HAPPINESS LEVEL:_____ALERTNESS LEVEL: _____

SUPPLIES NEEDED SOON: _____

MEDICATION TAKEN: _____

### NOTES

_____

_____

_____

# Activity & Caregiving Notes for _____ Date: _____

## TOILETING

| TIME | | | | | | | |
|------|--|--|--|--|--|--|--|
| U | | | | | | | |
| BM | | | | | | | |

### TIMES UP DURING THE NIGHT

_____  _____  _____  _____  _____

### TODAY I HAD A SHOWER/WASHED MY HAIR/SPONGE BATH

| Breakfast | |
|-----------|--|
| AM Snack | |
| Lunch | |
| PM Snack | |
| Dinner | |
| Drinks | |

### ACTIVITIES & OTHER COMMENTS

_____
_____
_____
_____
_____
_____

APPOINTMENTS: _____

HEALTH CONCERNS: _____

PLANS FOR TOMORROW: _____

PAIN LEVEL: _____HAPPINESS LEVEL:_____ALERTNESS LEVEL: _____

SUPPLIES NEEDED SOON:_____

MEDICATION TAKEN:_____

### NOTES

_____
_____
_____

# Activity & Caregiving Notes for _____ Date: _____

### TOILETING

| TIME | | | | | | | |
|------|--|--|--|--|--|--|--|
| U | | | | | | | |
| BM | | | | | | | |

### TIMES UP DURING THE NIGHT

_____    _____    _____    _____    _____

### TODAY I HAD A SHOWER/WASHED MY HAIR/SPONGE BATH

| Breakfast | |
|-----------|--|
| AM Snack | |
| Lunch | |
| PM Snack | |
| Dinner | |
| Drinks | |

### ACTIVITIES & OTHER COMMENTS

_____

_____

_____

_____

_____

_____

APPOINTMENTS: _____

HEALTH CONCERNS: _____

PLANS FOR TOMORROW: _____

PAIN LEVEL: _____HAPPINESS LEVEL:_____ALERTNESS LEVEL: _____

SUPPLIES NEEDED SOON: _____

MEDICATION TAKEN: _____

### NOTES

_____

_____

_____

# Activity & Caregiving Notes for _____ Date: _____

## TOILETING

| TIME | | | | | | | |
|------|---|---|---|---|---|---|---|
| U | | | | | | | |
| BM | | | | | | | |

### TIMES UP DURING THE NIGHT

_____   _____   _____   _____   _____

### TODAY I HAD A SHOWER/WASHED MY HAIR/SPONGE BATH

| Breakfast | |
|-----------|---|
| AM Snack | |
| Lunch | |
| PM Snack | |
| Dinner | |
| Drinks | |

### ACTIVITIES & OTHER COMMENTS

_____

_____

_____

_____

_____

_____

APPOINTMENTS: _____

HEALTH CONCERNS: _____

PLANS FOR TOMORROW: _____

PAIN LEVEL: _____ HAPPINESS LEVEL: _____ ALERTNESS LEVEL: _____

SUPPLIES NEEDED SOON: _____

MEDICATION TAKEN: _____

### NOTES

_____

_____

_____

# Activity & Caregiving Notes for _____ Date: _____

## TOILETING

| TIME | | | | | | | |
|------|---|---|---|---|---|---|---|
| U | | | | | | | |
| BM | | | | | | | |

### TIMES UP DURING THE NIGHT

_____   _____   _____   _____   _____

### TODAY I HAD A SHOWER/WASHED MY HAIR/SPONGE BATH

| Breakfast | |
|-----------|---|
| AM Snack | |
| Lunch | |
| PM Snack | |
| Dinner | |
| Drinks | |

### ACTIVITIES & OTHER COMMENTS

_____
_____
_____
_____
_____
_____

APPOINTMENTS: _____

HEALTH CONCERNS: _____

PLANS FOR TOMORROW: _____

PAIN LEVEL: _____ HAPPINESS LEVEL:_____ ALERTNESS LEVEL: _____

SUPPLIES NEEDED SOON:_____

MEDICATION TAKEN:_____

### NOTES

_____
_____
_____

# Activity & Caregiving Notes for _____ Date: _____

## TOILETING

| TIME | | | | | | | |
|------|--|--|--|--|--|--|--|
| **U** | | | | | | | |
| **BM** | | | | | | | |

### TIMES UP DURING THE NIGHT

_____  _____  _____  _____  _____

### TODAY I HAD A SHOWER/WASHED MY HAIR/SPONGE BATH

| Breakfast | |
|-----------|--|
| AM Snack | |
| Lunch | |
| PM Snack | |
| Dinner | |
| Drinks | |

### ACTIVITIES & OTHER COMMENTS

_____
_____
_____
_____
_____
_____

APPOINTMENTS: _____

HEALTH CONCERNS: _____

PLANS FOR TOMORROW: _____

PAIN LEVEL: _____ HAPPINESS LEVEL: _____ ALERTNESS LEVEL: _____

SUPPLIES NEEDED SOON: _____

MEDICATION TAKEN: _____

### NOTES

_____
_____
_____

# Activity & Caregiving Notes for _____ Date: _____

## TOILETING

| TIME | | | | | | | |
|------|--|--|--|--|--|--|--|
| U | | | | | | | |
| BM | | | | | | | |

### TIMES UP DURING THE NIGHT

_____  _____  _____  _____  _____

### TODAY I HAD A SHOWER/WASHED MY HAIR/SPONGE BATH

| Breakfast | |
|-----------|--|
| AM Snack | |
| Lunch | |
| PM Snack | |
| Dinner | |
| Drinks | |

### ACTIVITIES & OTHER COMMENTS

_____

_____

_____

_____

_____

_____

APPOINTMENTS: _____

HEALTH CONCERNS: _____

PLANS FOR TOMORROW: _____

PAIN LEVEL: _____HAPPINESS LEVEL:_____ALERTNESS LEVEL: _____

SUPPLIES NEEDED SOON: _____

MEDICATION TAKEN: _____

### NOTES

_____

_____

_____

# Activity & Caregiving Notes for _____ Date: _____

## TOILETING

| TIME | | | | | | | |
|------|--|--|--|--|--|--|--|
| U | | | | | | | |
| BM | | | | | | | |

TIMES UP DURING THE NIGHT

_____   _____   _____   _____   _____

TODAY I HAD A SHOWER/WASHED MY HAIR/SPONGE BATH

| Breakfast | |
|-----------|--|
| AM Snack | |
| Lunch | |
| PM Snack | |
| Dinner | |
| Drinks | |

## ACTIVITIES & OTHER COMMENTS

_____

_____

_____

_____

_____

_____

APPOINTMENTS: _____

HEALTH CONCERNS: _____

PLANS FOR TOMORROW: _____

PAIN LEVEL: _____ HAPPINESS LEVEL: _____ ALERTNESS LEVEL: _____

SUPPLIES NEEDED SOON: _____

MEDICATION TAKEN: _____

## NOTES

_____

_____

_____

# Activity & Caregiving Notes for _____ Date: _____

## TOILETING

| TIME | | | | | | | |
|------|---|---|---|---|---|---|---|
| U | | | | | | | |
| BM | | | | | | | |

### TIMES UP DURING THE NIGHT

_____   _____   _____   _____   _____

### TODAY I HAD A SHOWER/WASHED MY HAIR/SPONGE BATH

| Breakfast | |
|-----------|--|
| AM Snack | |
| Lunch | |
| PM Snack | |
| Dinner | |
| Drinks | |

### ACTIVITIES & OTHER COMMENTS

_____

_____

_____

_____

_____

_____

APPOINTMENTS: _____

HEALTH CONCERNS: _____

PLANS FOR TOMORROW: _____

PAIN LEVEL: _____ HAPPINESS LEVEL: _____ ALERTNESS LEVEL: _____

SUPPLIES NEEDED SOON: _____

MEDICATION TAKEN: _____

### NOTES

_____

_____

_____

# Activity & Caregiving Notes for _____ Date: _____

## TOILETING

| TIME | | | | | | | |
|------|--|--|--|--|--|--|--|
| U | | | | | | | |
| BM | | | | | | | |

### TIMES UP DURING THE NIGHT

_____    _____    _____    _____    _____

### TODAY I HAD A SHOWER/WASHED MY HAIR/SPONGE BATH

| Breakfast | |
|-----------|--|
| AM Snack | |
| Lunch | |
| PM Snack | |
| Dinner | |
| Drinks | |

### ACTIVITIES & OTHER COMMENTS

_____
_____
_____
_____
_____
_____

APPOINTMENTS: _____

HEALTH CONCERNS: _____

PLANS FOR TOMORROW: _____

PAIN LEVEL: _____ HAPPINESS LEVEL: _____ ALERTNESS LEVEL: _____

SUPPLIES NEEDED SOON: _____

MEDICATION TAKEN: _____

### NOTES

_____
_____
_____

# Activity & Caregiving Notes for _____ Date: _____

## TOILETING

| TIME | | | | | | | |
|------|--|--|--|--|--|--|--|
| U | | | | | | | |
| BM | | | | | | | |

TIMES UP DURING THE NIGHT

_____   _____   _____   _____   _____

TODAY I HAD A SHOWER/WASHED MY HAIR/SPONGE BATH

| Breakfast | |
|-----------|--|
| AM Snack | |
| Lunch | |
| PM Snack | |
| Dinner | |
| Drinks | |

## ACTIVITIES & OTHER COMMENTS

_____
_____
_____
_____
_____
_____
_____

APPOINTMENTS: _____
HEALTH CONCERNS: _____
PLANS FOR TOMORROW:_____
PAIN LEVEL: _____HAPPINESS LEVEL:_____ALERTNESS LEVEL: _____
SUPPLIES NEEDED SOON:_____
MEDICATION TAKEN:_____

## NOTES

_____
_____
_____

# Activity & Caregiving Notes for _____ Date: _____

## TOILETING

| TIME | | | | | | | |
|------|--|--|--|--|--|--|--|
| U | | | | | | | |
| BM | | | | | | | |

TIMES UP DURING THE NIGHT

_____  _____  _____  _____  _____

TODAY I HAD A SHOWER/WASHED MY HAIR/SPONGE BATH

| Breakfast | |
|-----------|--|
| AM Snack | |
| Lunch | |
| PM Snack | |
| Dinner | |
| Drinks | |

## ACTIVITIES & OTHER COMMENTS

_____

_____

_____

_____

_____

_____

APPOINTMENTS: _____

HEALTH CONCERNS: _____

PLANS FOR TOMORROW: _____

PAIN LEVEL: _____ HAPPINESS LEVEL: _____ ALERTNESS LEVEL: _____

SUPPLIES NEEDED SOON: _____

MEDICATION TAKEN: _____

## NOTES

_____

_____

_____

# Activity & Caregiving Notes for _____ Date: _____

## TOILETING

| TIME | | | | | | | |
|------|---|---|---|---|---|---|---|
| U | | | | | | | |
| BM | | | | | | | |

### TIMES UP DURING THE NIGHT

_____    _____    _____    _____    _____

### TODAY I HAD A SHOWER/WASHED MY HAIR/SPONGE BATH

| Breakfast | |
|-----------|---|
| AM Snack | |
| Lunch | |
| PM Snack | |
| Dinner | |
| Drinks | |

### ACTIVITIES & OTHER COMMENTS

_____

_____

_____

_____

_____

_____

APPOINTMENTS: _____

HEALTH CONCERNS: _____

PLANS FOR TOMORROW: _____

PAIN LEVEL: _____HAPPINESS LEVEL:_____ALERTNESS LEVEL: _____

SUPPLIES NEEDED SOON: _____

MEDICATION TAKEN: _____

### NOTES

_____

_____

_____

# Activity & Caregiving Notes for _____ Date: _____

## TOILETING

| TIME | | | | | | | |
|------|--|--|--|--|--|--|--|
| U | | | | | | | |
| BM | | | | | | | |

TIMES UP DURING THE NIGHT

_____  _____  _____  _____  _____

TODAY I HAD A SHOWER/WASHED MY HAIR/SPONGE BATH

| Breakfast | |
|-----------|--|
| AM Snack | |
| Lunch | |
| PM Snack | |
| Dinner | |
| Drinks | |

## ACTIVITIES & OTHER COMMENTS

_____

_____

_____

_____

_____

_____

APPOINTMENTS: _____

HEALTH CONCERNS: _____

PLANS FOR TOMORROW:_____

PAIN LEVEL: _____HAPPINESS LEVEL:_____ALERTNESS LEVEL: _____

SUPPLIES NEEDED SOON:_____

MEDICATION TAKEN:_____

## NOTES

_____

_____

_____

# Activity & Caregiving Notes for _____ Date: _____

## TOILETING

| TIME | | | | | | | |
|------|---|---|---|---|---|---|---|
| U | | | | | | | |
| BM | | | | | | | |

### TIMES UP DURING THE NIGHT

_____ _____ _____ _____ _____

### TODAY I HAD A SHOWER/WASHED MY HAIR/SPONGE BATH

| Breakfast | |
|-----------|---|
| AM Snack | |
| Lunch | |
| PM Snack | |
| Dinner | |
| Drinks | |

### ACTIVITIES & OTHER COMMENTS

_____
_____
_____
_____
_____
_____

APPOINTMENTS: _____

HEALTH CONCERNS: _____

PLANS FOR TOMORROW: _____

PAIN LEVEL: _____ HAPPINESS LEVEL: _____ ALERTNESS LEVEL: _____

SUPPLIES NEEDED SOON: _____

MEDICATION TAKEN: _____

### NOTES

_____
_____
_____

# Activity & Caregiving Notes for _____ Date: _____

## TOILETING

| TIME | | | | | | | |
|------|--|--|--|--|--|--|--|
| U | | | | | | | |
| BM | | | | | | | |

### TIMES UP DURING THE NIGHT

_____    _____    _____    _____    _____

### TODAY I HAD A SHOWER/WASHED MY HAIR/SPONGE BATH

| Breakfast | |
|-----------|--|
| AM Snack | |
| Lunch | |
| PM Snack | |
| Dinner | |
| Drinks | |

### ACTIVITIES & OTHER COMMENTS

_____
_____
_____
_____
_____
_____

APPOINTMENTS: _____

HEALTH CONCERNS: _____

PLANS FOR TOMORROW: _____

PAIN LEVEL: _____ HAPPINESS LEVEL: _____ ALERTNESS LEVEL: _____

SUPPLIES NEEDED SOON: _____

MEDICATION TAKEN: _____

### NOTES

_____
_____
_____

# Activity & Caregiving Notes for _____ Date: _____

## TOILETING

| TIME | | | | | | | |
|------|--|--|--|--|--|--|--|
| U    | | | | | | | |
| BM   | | | | | | | |

TIMES UP DURING THE NIGHT

_____  _____  _____  _____  _____

TODAY I HAD A SHOWER/WASHED MY HAIR/SPONGE BATH

| Breakfast | |
|-----------|--|
| AM Snack  | |
| Lunch     | |
| PM Snack  | |
| Dinner    | |
| Drinks    | |

## ACTIVITIES & OTHER COMMENTS

_____

_____

_____

_____

_____

_____

APPOINTMENTS: _____

HEALTH CONCERNS: _____

PLANS FOR TOMORROW: _____

PAIN LEVEL: _____ HAPPINESS LEVEL: _____ ALERTNESS LEVEL: _____

SUPPLIES NEEDED SOON: _____

MEDICATION TAKEN: _____

## NOTES

_____

_____

_____

# Activity & Caregiving Notes for _____ Date: _____

## TOILETING

| TIME | | | | | | | |
|------|--|--|--|--|--|--|--|
| U | | | | | | | |
| BM | | | | | | | |

### TIMES UP DURING THE NIGHT

_____   _____   _____   _____   _____

### TODAY I HAD A SHOWER/WASHED MY HAIR/SPONGE BATH

| Breakfast | |
|-----------|--|
| AM Snack | |
| Lunch | |
| PM Snack | |
| Dinner | |
| Drinks | |

### ACTIVITIES & OTHER COMMENTS

_____

_____

_____

_____

_____

_____

APPOINTMENTS: _____

HEALTH CONCERNS: _____

PLANS FOR TOMORROW: _____

PAIN LEVEL: _____ HAPPINESS LEVEL: _____ ALERTNESS LEVEL: _____

SUPPLIES NEEDED SOON: _____

MEDICATION TAKEN: _____

### NOTES

_____

_____

_____

# Activity & Caregiving Notes for _____ Date: _____

## TOILETING

| TIME | | | | | | | |
|------|---|---|---|---|---|---|---|
| U | | | | | | | |
| BM | | | | | | | |

### TIMES UP DURING THE NIGHT

_____  _____  _____  _____  _____

### TODAY I HAD A SHOWER/WASHED MY HAIR/SPONGE BATH

| Breakfast | |
|-----------|---|
| AM Snack | |
| Lunch | |
| PM Snack | |
| Dinner | |
| Drinks | |

### ACTIVITIES & OTHER COMMENTS

_____

_____

_____

_____

_____

_____

APPOINTMENTS: _____

HEALTH CONCERNS: _____

PLANS FOR TOMORROW: _____

PAIN LEVEL: _____ HAPPINESS LEVEL: _____ ALERTNESS LEVEL: _____

SUPPLIES NEEDED SOON: _____

MEDICATION TAKEN: _____

### NOTES

_____

_____

_____

# Activity & Caregiving Notes for _____ Date: _____

## TOILETING

| TIME | | | | | | | |
|------|---|---|---|---|---|---|---|
| U | | | | | | | |
| BM | | | | | | | |

### TIMES UP DURING THE NIGHT

_____  _____  _____  _____  _____

### TODAY I HAD A SHOWER/WASHED MY HAIR/SPONGE BATH

| Breakfast | |
|-----------|---|
| AM Snack | |
| Lunch | |
| PM Snack | |
| Dinner | |
| Drinks | |

### ACTIVITIES & OTHER COMMENTS

_____
_____
_____
_____
_____
_____

APPOINTMENTS: _____

HEALTH CONCERNS: _____

PLANS FOR TOMORROW: _____

PAIN LEVEL: _____ HAPPINESS LEVEL: _____ ALERTNESS LEVEL: _____

SUPPLIES NEEDED SOON: _____

MEDICATION TAKEN: _____

### NOTES

_____
_____
_____

# Activity & Caregiving Notes for _____ Date: _____

## TOILETING

| TIME | | | | | | | | |
|------|--|--|--|--|--|--|--|--|
| U | | | | | | | | |
| BM | | | | | | | | |

### TIMES UP DURING THE NIGHT

_____    _____    _____    _____    _____

### TODAY I HAD A SHOWER/WASHED MY HAIR/SPONGE BATH

| Breakfast | |
|-----------|--|
| AM Snack | |
| Lunch | |
| PM Snack | |
| Dinner | |
| Drinks | |

### ACTIVITIES & OTHER COMMENTS

_____
_____
_____
_____
_____
_____

APPOINTMENTS: _____
HEALTH CONCERNS: _____
PLANS FOR TOMORROW: _____
PAIN LEVEL: _____ HAPPINESS LEVEL: _____ ALERTNESS LEVEL: _____
SUPPLIES NEEDED SOON: _____
MEDICATION TAKEN: _____

### NOTES

_____
_____
_____

# Activity & Caregiving Notes for _____ Date: _____

## TOILETING

| TIME | | | | | | | |
|------|--|--|--|--|--|--|--|
| U | | | | | | | |
| BM | | | | | | | |

### TIMES UP DURING THE NIGHT

_____  _____  _____  _____  _____

### TODAY I HAD A SHOWER/WASHED MY HAIR/SPONGE BATH

| Breakfast | |
|-----------|--|
| AM Snack | |
| Lunch | |
| PM Snack | |
| Dinner | |
| Drinks | |

### ACTIVITIES & OTHER COMMENTS

_____
_____
_____
_____
_____
_____

APPOINTMENTS: _____

HEALTH CONCERNS: _____

PLANS FOR TOMORROW: _____

PAIN LEVEL: _____ HAPPINESS LEVEL: _____ ALERTNESS LEVEL: _____

SUPPLIES NEEDED SOON: _____

MEDICATION TAKEN: _____

### NOTES

_____
_____
_____

# Activity & Caregiving Notes for _____ Date: _____

### TOILETING

| TIME | | | | | | | |
|------|--|--|--|--|--|--|--|
| U | | | | | | | |
| BM | | | | | | | |

TIMES UP DURING THE NIGHT

_____    _____    _____    _____    _____

TODAY I HAD A SHOWER/WASHED MY HAIR/SPONGE BATH

| Breakfast | |
|-----------|--|
| AM Snack | |
| Lunch | |
| PM Snack | |
| Dinner | |
| Drinks | |

### ACTIVITIES & OTHER COMMENTS

_____

_____

_____

_____

_____

_____

APPOINTMENTS: _____

HEALTH CONCERNS: _____

PLANS FOR TOMORROW: _____

PAIN LEVEL: _____ HAPPINESS LEVEL: _____ ALERTNESS LEVEL: _____

SUPPLIES NEEDED SOON: _____

MEDICATION TAKEN: _____

### NOTES

_____

_____

_____

# Activity & Caregiving Notes for _____ Date: _____

## TOILETING

| TIME | | | | | | | |
|------|--|--|--|--|--|--|--|
| U | | | | | | | |
| BM | | | | | | | |

### TIMES UP DURING THE NIGHT

_____   _____   _____   _____   _____

### TODAY I HAD A SHOWER/WASHED MY HAIR/SPONGE BATH

| Breakfast | |
|-----------|--|
| AM Snack | |
| Lunch | |
| PM Snack | |
| Dinner | |
| Drinks | |

### ACTIVITIES & OTHER COMMENTS

_____

_____

_____

_____

_____

_____

APPOINTMENTS: _____

HEALTH CONCERNS: _____

PLANS FOR TOMORROW: _____

PAIN LEVEL: _____ HAPPINESS LEVEL: _____ ALERTNESS LEVEL: _____

SUPPLIES NEEDED SOON: _____

MEDICATION TAKEN: _____

### NOTES

_____

_____

_____

# Activity & Caregiving Notes for _____ Date: _____

### TOILETING

| TIME | | | | | | | |
|------|--|--|--|--|--|--|--|
| U | | | | | | | |
| BM | | | | | | | |

### TIMES UP DURING THE NIGHT

_____   _____   _____   _____   _____

### TODAY I HAD A SHOWER/WASHED MY HAIR/SPONGE BATH

| Breakfast | |
|-----------|--|
| AM Snack | |
| Lunch | |
| PM Snack | |
| Dinner | |
| Drinks | |

### ACTIVITIES & OTHER COMMENTS

_____
_____
_____
_____
_____
_____

APPOINTMENTS: _____
HEALTH CONCERNS: _____
PLANS FOR TOMORROW: _____
PAIN LEVEL: _____ HAPPINESS LEVEL: _____ ALERTNESS LEVEL: _____
SUPPLIES NEEDED SOON: _____
MEDICATION TAKEN: _____

### NOTES

_____
_____
_____

# Activity & Caregiving Notes for _____ Date: _____

## TOILETING

| TIME | | | | | | | |
|------|--|--|--|--|--|--|--|
| U | | | | | | | |
| BM | | | | | | | |

TIMES UP DURING THE NIGHT

_____   _____   _____   _____   _____

TODAY I HAD A SHOWER/WASHED MY HAIR/SPONGE BATH

| Breakfast | |
|-----------|--|
| AM Snack | |
| Lunch | |
| PM Snack | |
| Dinner | |
| Drinks | |

## ACTIVITIES & OTHER COMMENTS

_____
_____
_____
_____
_____
_____

APPOINTMENTS: _____
HEALTH CONCERNS: _____
PLANS FOR TOMORROW: _____
PAIN LEVEL: _____ HAPPINESS LEVEL: _____ ALERTNESS LEVEL: _____
SUPPLIES NEEDED SOON: _____
MEDICATION TAKEN: _____

## NOTES

_____
_____
_____

# Activity & Caregiving Notes for _____ Date: _____

## TOILETING

| TIME | | | | | | | |
|------|--|--|--|--|--|--|--|
| U | | | | | | | |
| BM | | | | | | | |

### TIMES UP DURING THE NIGHT

_____ _____ _____ _____ _____

### TODAY I HAD A SHOWER/WASHED MY HAIR/SPONGE BATH

| Breakfast | |
|-----------|--|
| AM Snack | |
| Lunch | |
| PM Snack | |
| Dinner | |
| Drinks | |

### ACTIVITIES & OTHER COMMENTS

_____

_____

_____

_____

_____

_____

APPOINTMENTS: _____

HEALTH CONCERNS: _____

PLANS FOR TOMORROW: _____

PAIN LEVEL: _____ HAPPINESS LEVEL: _____ ALERTNESS LEVEL: _____

SUPPLIES NEEDED SOON: _____

MEDICATION TAKEN: _____

### NOTES

_____

_____

_____

# Activity & Caregiving Notes for _____ Date: _____

### TOILETING

| TIME | | | | | | | |
|------|--|--|--|--|--|--|--|
| U | | | | | | | |
| BM | | | | | | | |

### TIMES UP DURING THE NIGHT

_____   _____   _____   _____   _____

### TODAY I HAD A SHOWER/WASHED MY HAIR/SPONGE BATH

| Breakfast | |
|-----------|--|
| AM Snack | |
| Lunch | |
| PM Snack | |
| Dinner | |
| Drinks | |

### ACTIVITIES & OTHER COMMENTS

_____
_____
_____
_____
_____
_____

APPOINTMENTS: _____

HEALTH CONCERNS: _____

PLANS FOR TOMORROW: _____

PAIN LEVEL: _____ HAPPINESS LEVEL: _____ ALERTNESS LEVEL: _____

SUPPLIES NEEDED SOON: _____

MEDICATION TAKEN: _____

### NOTES

_____
_____
_____

# Activity & Caregiving Notes for _____ Date: _____

## TOILETING

| TIME | | | | | | | |
|------|--|--|--|--|--|--|--|
| U | | | | | | | |
| BM | | | | | | | |

### TIMES UP DURING THE NIGHT

_____   _____   _____   _____   _____

### TODAY I HAD A SHOWER/WASHED MY HAIR/SPONGE BATH

| Breakfast | |
|-----------|--|
| AM Snack | |
| Lunch | |
| PM Snack | |
| Dinner | |
| Drinks | |

### ACTIVITIES & OTHER COMMENTS

_____
_____
_____
_____
_____
_____

APPOINTMENTS: _____
HEALTH CONCERNS: _____
PLANS FOR TOMORROW: _____
PAIN LEVEL: _____ HAPPINESS LEVEL: _____ ALERTNESS LEVEL: _____
SUPPLIES NEEDED SOON: _____
MEDICATION TAKEN: _____

### NOTES

_____
_____
_____

# Activity & Caregiving Notes for _____ Date: _____

### TOILETING

| TIME | | | | | | | |
|------|--|--|--|--|--|--|--|
| U | | | | | | | |
| BM | | | | | | | |

### TIMES UP DURING THE NIGHT

_____ _____ _____ _____ _____

### TODAY I HAD A SHOWER/WASHED MY HAIR/SPONGE BATH

| Breakfast | |
|-----------|--|
| AM Snack | |
| Lunch | |
| PM Snack | |
| Dinner | |
| Drinks | |

### ACTIVITIES & OTHER COMMENTS

_____
_____
_____
_____
_____
_____

APPOINTMENTS: _____

HEALTH CONCERNS: _____

PLANS FOR TOMORROW:_____

PAIN LEVEL: _____HAPPINESS LEVEL:_____ALERTNESS LEVEL: _____

SUPPLIES NEEDED SOON:_____

MEDICATION TAKEN:_____

### NOTES

_____
_____
_____

# Activity & Caregiving Notes for _____ Date: _____

## TOILETING

| TIME | | | | | | | |
|------|---|---|---|---|---|---|---|
| U | | | | | | | |
| BM | | | | | | | |

TIMES UP DURING THE NIGHT

_____   _____   _____   _____   _____

TODAY I HAD A SHOWER/WASHED MY HAIR/SPONGE BATH

| Breakfast | |
|-----------|---|
| AM Snack | |
| Lunch | |
| PM Snack | |
| Dinner | |
| Drinks | |

## ACTIVITIES & OTHER COMMENTS

_____

_____

_____

_____

_____

_____

APPOINTMENTS: _____

HEALTH CONCERNS: _____

PLANS FOR TOMORROW:_____

PAIN LEVEL: _____HAPPINESS LEVEL:_____ALERTNESS LEVEL: _____

SUPPLIES NEEDED SOON:_____

MEDICATION TAKEN:_____

## NOTES

_____

_____

_____

# Activity & Caregiving Notes for _____ Date: _____

## TOILETING

| TIME | | | | | | | |
|------|--|--|--|--|--|--|--|
| U | | | | | | | |
| BM | | | | | | | |

### TIMES UP DURING THE NIGHT

_____  _____  _____  _____  _____

### TODAY I HAD A SHOWER/WASHED MY HAIR/SPONGE BATH

| Breakfast | |
|-----------|--|
| AM Snack | |
| Lunch | |
| PM Snack | |
| Dinner | |
| Drinks | |

### ACTIVITIES & OTHER COMMENTS

_____
_____
_____
_____
_____
_____

APPOINTMENTS: _____
HEALTH CONCERNS: _____
PLANS FOR TOMORROW: _____
PAIN LEVEL: _____ HAPPINESS LEVEL: _____ ALERTNESS LEVEL: _____
SUPPLIES NEEDED SOON: _____
MEDICATION TAKEN: _____

### NOTES

_____
_____
_____

# Activity & Caregiving Notes for _____ Date: _____

## TOILETING

| TIME | | | | | | | |
|------|---|---|---|---|---|---|---|
| U | | | | | | | |
| BM | | | | | | | |

TIMES UP DURING THE NIGHT

_____   _____   _____   _____   _____

TODAY I HAD A SHOWER/WASHED MY HAIR/SPONGE BATH

| Breakfast | |
|-----------|---|
| AM Snack | |
| Lunch | |
| PM Snack | |
| Dinner | |
| Drinks | |

## ACTIVITIES & OTHER COMMENTS

_____

_____

_____

_____

_____

_____

APPOINTMENTS: _____

HEALTH CONCERNS: _____

PLANS FOR TOMORROW: _____

PAIN LEVEL: _____HAPPINESS LEVEL:_____ALERTNESS LEVEL: _____

SUPPLIES NEEDED SOON: _____

MEDICATION TAKEN: _____

## NOTES

_____

_____

_____

# Activity & Caregiving Notes for _____ Date: _____

## TOILETING

| TIME | | | | | | | |
|------|---|---|---|---|---|---|---|
| U | | | | | | | |
| BM | | | | | | | |

### TIMES UP DURING THE NIGHT

_____   _____   _____   _____   _____

### TODAY I HAD A SHOWER/WASHED MY HAIR/SPONGE BATH

| Breakfast | |
|-----------|---|
| AM Snack | |
| Lunch | |
| PM Snack | |
| Dinner | |
| Drinks | |

### ACTIVITIES & OTHER COMMENTS

_____

_____

_____

_____

_____

_____

APPOINTMENTS: _____

HEALTH CONCERNS: _____

PLANS FOR TOMORROW: _____

PAIN LEVEL: _____HAPPINESS LEVEL:_____ALERTNESS LEVEL: _____

SUPPLIES NEEDED SOON:_____

MEDICATION TAKEN:_____

### NOTES

_____

_____

_____

# Activity & Caregiving Notes for _____ Date: _____

## TOILETING

| TIME | | | | | | | |
|------|--|--|--|--|--|--|--|
| U | | | | | | | |
| BM | | | | | | | |

TIMES UP DURING THE NIGHT

_____   _____   _____   _____   _____

TODAY I HAD A SHOWER/WASHED MY HAIR/SPONGE BATH

| Breakfast | |
|-----------|--|
| AM Snack | |
| Lunch | |
| PM Snack | |
| Dinner | |
| Drinks | |

## ACTIVITIES & OTHER COMMENTS

_____
_____
_____
_____
_____
_____

APPOINTMENTS: _____
HEALTH CONCERNS: _____
PLANS FOR TOMORROW:_____
PAIN LEVEL: _____HAPPINESS LEVEL:_____ALERTNESS LEVEL: _____
SUPPLIES NEEDED SOON:_____
MEDICATION TAKEN:_____

## NOTES

_____
_____
_____

# Activity & Caregiving Notes for _____ Date: _____

## TOILETING

| TIME | | | | | | | |
|------|---|---|---|---|---|---|---|
| U | | | | | | | |
| BM | | | | | | | |

TIMES UP DURING THE NIGHT

_____  _____  _____  _____  _____

TODAY I HAD A SHOWER/WASHED MY HAIR/SPONGE BATH

| Breakfast | |
|-----------|---|
| AM Snack | |
| Lunch | |
| PM Snack | |
| Dinner | |
| Drinks | |

ACTIVITIES & OTHER COMMENTS

_____
_____
_____
_____
_____
_____

APPOINTMENTS: _____
HEALTH CONCERNS: _____
PLANS FOR TOMORROW: _____
PAIN LEVEL: _____ HAPPINESS LEVEL:_____ ALERTNESS LEVEL: _____
SUPPLIES NEEDED SOON: _____
MEDICATION TAKEN: _____

NOTES

_____
_____
_____

# Activity & Caregiving Notes for _____ Date: _____

## TOILETING

| TIME | | | | | | | |
|------|---|---|---|---|---|---|---|
| U | | | | | | | |
| BM | | | | | | | |

### TIMES UP DURING THE NIGHT

_____     _____     _____     _____     _____

### TODAY I HAD A SHOWER/WASHED MY HAIR/SPONGE BATH

| Breakfast | |
|-----------|---|
| AM Snack | |
| Lunch | |
| PM Snack | |
| Dinner | |
| Drinks | |

### ACTIVITIES & OTHER COMMENTS

_____

_____

_____

_____

_____

_____

APPOINTMENTS: _____

HEALTH CONCERNS: _____

PLANS FOR TOMORROW: _____

PAIN LEVEL: _____ HAPPINESS LEVEL: _____ ALERTNESS LEVEL: _____

SUPPLIES NEEDED SOON: _____

MEDICATION TAKEN: _____

### NOTES

_____

_____

_____

# Activity & Caregiving Notes for _____ Date: _____

## TOILETING

| TIME | | | | | | | |
|---|---|---|---|---|---|---|---|
| U | | | | | | | |
| BM | | | | | | | |

### TIMES UP DURING THE NIGHT

_____  _____  _____  _____  _____

### TODAY I HAD A SHOWER/WASHED MY HAIR/SPONGE BATH

| Breakfast | |
|---|---|
| AM Snack | |
| Lunch | |
| PM Snack | |
| Dinner | |
| Drinks | |

### ACTIVITIES & OTHER COMMENTS

_____
_____
_____
_____
_____
_____

APPOINTMENTS: _____
HEALTH CONCERNS: _____
PLANS FOR TOMORROW: _____
PAIN LEVEL: _____ HAPPINESS LEVEL: _____ ALERTNESS LEVEL: _____
SUPPLIES NEEDED SOON: _____
MEDICATION TAKEN: _____

### NOTES

_____
_____
_____

# Activity & Caregiving Notes for _____ Date: _____

### TOILETING

| TIME | | | | | | | |
|------|---|---|---|---|---|---|---|
| U | | | | | | | |
| BM | | | | | | | |

### TIMES UP DURING THE NIGHT

_____    _____    _____    _____    _____

### TODAY I HAD A SHOWER/WASHED MY HAIR/SPONGE BATH

| Breakfast | |
|-----------|---|
| AM Snack | |
| Lunch | |
| PM Snack | |
| Dinner | |
| Drinks | |

### ACTIVITIES & OTHER COMMENTS

_____

_____

_____

_____

_____

_____

APPOINTMENTS: _____

HEALTH CONCERNS: _____

PLANS FOR TOMORROW: _____

PAIN LEVEL: _____ HAPPINESS LEVEL: _____ ALERTNESS LEVEL: _____

SUPPLIES NEEDED SOON: _____

MEDICATION TAKEN: _____

### NOTES

_____

_____

_____

# Activity & Caregiving Notes for _____ Date: _____

## TOILETING

| TIME | | | | | | | |
|------|--|--|--|--|--|--|--|
| U | | | | | | | |
| BM | | | | | | | |

TIMES UP DURING THE NIGHT

_____    _____    _____    _____    _____

TODAY I HAD A SHOWER/WASHED MY HAIR/SPONGE BATH

| Breakfast | |
|-----------|--|
| AM Snack | |
| Lunch | |
| PM Snack | |
| Dinner | |
| Drinks | |

## ACTIVITIES & OTHER COMMENTS

_____

_____

_____

_____

_____

_____

APPOINTMENTS: _____

HEALTH CONCERNS: _____

PLANS FOR TOMORROW: _____

PAIN LEVEL: _____HAPPINESS LEVEL:_____ALERTNESS LEVEL: _____

SUPPLIES NEEDED SOON:_____

MEDICATION TAKEN:_____

## NOTES

_____

_____

_____

# Activity & Caregiving Notes for _____ Date: _____

### TOILETING

| TIME | | | | | | | |
|------|--|--|--|--|--|--|--|
| U | | | | | | | |
| BM | | | | | | | |

### TIMES UP DURING THE NIGHT

_____    _____    _____    _____    _____

### TODAY I HAD A SHOWER/WASHED MY HAIR/SPONGE BATH

| Breakfast | |
|-----------|--|
| AM Snack | |
| Lunch | |
| PM Snack | |
| Dinner | |
| Drinks | |

### ACTIVITIES & OTHER COMMENTS

_____

_____

_____

_____

_____

_____

APPOINTMENTS: _____

HEALTH CONCERNS: _____

PLANS FOR TOMORROW: _____

PAIN LEVEL: _____HAPPINESS LEVEL:_____ALERTNESS LEVEL: _____

SUPPLIES NEEDED SOON: _____

MEDICATION TAKEN:_____

### NOTES

_____

_____

_____

# Activity & Caregiving Notes for _____ Date: _____

## TOILETING

| TIME | | | | | | | |
|------|--|--|--|--|--|--|--|
| U | | | | | | | |
| BM | | | | | | | |

### TIMES UP DURING THE NIGHT

_____  _____  _____  _____  _____

### TODAY I HAD A SHOWER/WASHED MY HAIR/SPONGE BATH

| Breakfast | |
|-----------|--|
| AM Snack | |
| Lunch | |
| PM Snack | |
| Dinner | |
| Drinks | |

### ACTIVITIES & OTHER COMMENTS

_____
_____
_____
_____
_____
_____

APPOINTMENTS: _____
HEALTH CONCERNS: _____
PLANS FOR TOMORROW: _____
PAIN LEVEL: _____ HAPPINESS LEVEL: _____ ALERTNESS LEVEL: _____
SUPPLIES NEEDED SOON: _____
MEDICATION TAKEN: _____

### NOTES

_____
_____
_____

# Activity & Caregiving Notes for _____ Date: _____

## TOILETING

| TIME | | | | | | | |
|------|--|--|--|--|--|--|--|
| U | | | | | | | |
| BM | | | | | | | |

### TIMES UP DURING THE NIGHT

_____   _____   _____   _____   _____

### TODAY I HAD A SHOWER/WASHED MY HAIR/SPONGE BATH

| Breakfast | |
|-----------|--|
| AM Snack | |
| Lunch | |
| PM Snack | |
| Dinner | |
| Drinks | |

### ACTIVITIES & OTHER COMMENTS

_____

_____

_____

_____

_____

_____

APPOINTMENTS: _____

HEALTH CONCERNS: _____

PLANS FOR TOMORROW: _____

PAIN LEVEL: _____HAPPINESS LEVEL:_____ALERTNESS LEVEL: _____

SUPPLIES NEEDED SOON: _____

MEDICATION TAKEN:_____

### NOTES

_____

_____

_____

# Activity & Caregiving Notes for _____ Date: _____

## TOILETING

| TIME | | | | | | | |
|------|--|--|--|--|--|--|--|
| U | | | | | | | |
| BM | | | | | | | |

TIMES UP DURING THE NIGHT

_____   _____   _____   _____   _____

TODAY I HAD A SHOWER/WASHED MY HAIR/SPONGE BATH

| Breakfast | |
|-----------|--|
| AM Snack | |
| Lunch | |
| PM Snack | |
| Dinner | |
| Drinks | |

## ACTIVITIES & OTHER COMMENTS

_____

_____

_____

_____

_____

_____

APPOINTMENTS: _____

HEALTH CONCERNS: _____

PLANS FOR TOMORROW: _____

PAIN LEVEL: _____ HAPPINESS LEVEL: _____ ALERTNESS LEVEL: _____

SUPPLIES NEEDED SOON: _____

MEDICATION TAKEN: _____

## NOTES

_____

_____

_____

# Activity & Caregiving Notes for _____ Date: ____

### TOILETING

| TIME | | | | | | | |
|------|---|---|---|---|---|---|---|
| U | | | | | | | |
| BM | | | | | | | |

### TIMES UP DURING THE NIGHT

_____   _____   _____   _____   _____

### TODAY I HAD A SHOWER/WASHED MY HAIR/SPONGE BATH

| Breakfast | |
|-----------|---|
| AM Snack | |
| Lunch | |
| PM Snack | |
| Dinner | |
| Drinks | |

### ACTIVITIES & OTHER COMMENTS

_____

_____

_____

_____

_____

_____

APPOINTMENTS: _____

HEALTH CONCERNS: _____

PLANS FOR TOMORROW: _____

PAIN LEVEL: _____ HAPPINESS LEVEL: _____ ALERTNESS LEVEL: _____

SUPPLIES NEEDED SOON: _____

MEDICATION TAKEN: _____

### NOTES

_____

_____

_____

# Activity & Caregiving Notes for _____ Date: _____

## TOILETING

| TIME | | | | | | | |
|------|--|--|--|--|--|--|--|
| **U** | | | | | | | |
| **BM** | | | | | | | |

### TIMES UP DURING THE NIGHT

_____   _____   _____   _____   _____

### TODAY I HAD A SHOWER/WASHED MY HAIR/SPONGE BATH

| Breakfast | |
|-----------|--|
| AM Snack | |
| Lunch | |
| PM Snack | |
| Dinner | |
| Drinks | |

### ACTIVITIES & OTHER COMMENTS

_____
_____
_____
_____
_____
_____

APPOINTMENTS: _____

HEALTH CONCERNS: _____

PLANS FOR TOMORROW: _____

PAIN LEVEL: _____ HAPPINESS LEVEL: _____ ALERTNESS LEVEL: _____

SUPPLIES NEEDED SOON: _____

MEDICATION TAKEN: _____

### NOTES

_____
_____
_____

# Activity & Caregiving Notes for _____ Date: _____

## TOILETING

| TIME | | | | | | | |
|------|---|---|---|---|---|---|---|
| U | | | | | | | |
| BM | | | | | | | |

### TIMES UP DURING THE NIGHT

_____    _____    _____    _____    _____

### TODAY I HAD A SHOWER/WASHED MY HAIR/SPONGE BATH

| Breakfast | |
|-----------|---|
| AM Snack | |
| Lunch | |
| PM Snack | |
| Dinner | |
| Drinks | |

### ACTIVITIES & OTHER COMMENTS

_____

_____

_____

_____

_____

_____

APPOINTMENTS: _____

HEALTH CONCERNS: _____

PLANS FOR TOMORROW: _____

PAIN LEVEL: _____ HAPPINESS LEVEL: _____ ALERTNESS LEVEL: _____

SUPPLIES NEEDED SOON: _____

MEDICATION TAKEN: _____

### NOTES

_____

_____

_____

# Activity & Caregiving Notes for _____ Date: _____

## TOILETING

| TIME | | | | | | | |
|------|---|---|---|---|---|---|---|
| U | | | | | | | |
| BM | | | | | | | |

### TIMES UP DURING THE NIGHT

_____  _____  _____  _____  _____

### TODAY I HAD A SHOWER/WASHED MY HAIR/SPONGE BATH

| Breakfast | |
|-----------|---|
| AM Snack | |
| Lunch | |
| PM Snack | |
| Dinner | |
| Drinks | |

### ACTIVITIES & OTHER COMMENTS

_____

_____

_____

_____

_____

_____

APPOINTMENTS: _____

HEALTH CONCERNS: _____

PLANS FOR TOMORROW: _____

PAIN LEVEL: _____ HAPPINESS LEVEL: _____ ALERTNESS LEVEL: _____

SUPPLIES NEEDED SOON: _____

MEDICATION TAKEN: _____

### NOTES

_____

_____

_____

# Activity & Caregiving Notes for _____ Date: _____

## TOILETING

| TIME | | | | | | | |
|------|---|---|---|---|---|---|---|
| U | | | | | | | |
| BM | | | | | | | |

### TIMES UP DURING THE NIGHT

_____    _____    _____    _____    _____

### TODAY I HAD A SHOWER/WASHED MY HAIR/SPONGE BATH

| Breakfast | |
|-----------|---|
| AM Snack | |
| Lunch | |
| PM Snack | |
| Dinner | |
| Drinks | |

### ACTIVITIES & OTHER COMMENTS

_____

_____

_____

_____

_____

_____

APPOINTMENTS: _____

HEALTH CONCERNS: _____

PLANS FOR TOMORROW: _____

PAIN LEVEL: _____ HAPPINESS LEVEL: _____ ALERTNESS LEVEL: _____

SUPPLIES NEEDED SOON: _____

MEDICATION TAKEN: _____

### NOTES

_____

_____

_____

# Activity & Caregiving Notes for _____ Date: _____

TOILETING

| TIME | | | | | | | |
|------|---|---|---|---|---|---|---|
| U | | | | | | | |
| BM | | | | | | | |

TIMES UP DURING THE NIGHT

_____   _____   _____   _____   _____

TODAY I HAD A SHOWER/WASHED MY HAIR/SPONGE BATH

| Breakfast | |
|-----------|---|
| AM Snack | |
| Lunch | |
| PM Snack | |
| Dinner | |
| Drinks | |

ACTIVITIES & OTHER COMMENTS

_____

_____

_____

_____

_____

_____

APPOINTMENTS: _____

HEALTH CONCERNS: _____

PLANS FOR TOMORROW: _____

PAIN LEVEL: _____HAPPINESS LEVEL:_____ALERTNESS LEVEL: _____

SUPPLIES NEEDED SOON: _____

MEDICATION TAKEN: _____

NOTES

_____

_____

_____

# Activity & Caregiving Notes for _____ Date: _____

### TOILETING

| TIME | | | | | | | |
|------|--|--|--|--|--|--|--|
| U | | | | | | | |
| BM | | | | | | | |

### TIMES UP DURING THE NIGHT

_____   _____   _____   _____   _____

### TODAY I HAD A SHOWER/WASHED MY HAIR/SPONGE BATH

| Breakfast | |
|-----------|--|
| AM Snack | |
| Lunch | |
| PM Snack | |
| Dinner | |
| Drinks | |

### ACTIVITIES & OTHER COMMENTS

_____

_____

_____

_____

_____

_____

APPOINTMENTS: _____

HEALTH CONCERNS: _____

PLANS FOR TOMORROW: _____

PAIN LEVEL: _____HAPPINESS LEVEL:_____ALERTNESS LEVEL: _____

SUPPLIES NEEDED SOON: _____

MEDICATION TAKEN: _____

### NOTES

_____

_____

_____

# Activity & Caregiving Notes for _____ Date: _____

### TOILETING

| TIME | | | | | | | |
|------|---|---|---|---|---|---|---|
| U    | | | | | | | |
| BM   | | | | | | | |

### TIMES UP DURING THE NIGHT

_____  _____  _____  _____  _____

### TODAY I HAD A SHOWER/WASHED MY HAIR/SPONGE BATH

| Breakfast | |
|-----------|---|
| AM Snack  | |
| Lunch     | |
| PM Snack  | |
| Dinner    | |
| Drinks    | |

### ACTIVITIES & OTHER COMMENTS

_____

_____

_____

_____

_____

_____

APPOINTMENTS: _____

HEALTH CONCERNS: _____

PLANS FOR TOMORROW: _____

PAIN LEVEL: _____ HAPPINESS LEVEL: _____ ALERTNESS LEVEL: _____

SUPPLIES NEEDED SOON: _____

MEDICATION TAKEN: _____

### NOTES

_____

_____

_____

# Activity & Caregiving Notes for _____ Date: _____

### TOILETING

| TIME | | | | | | | |
|------|--|--|--|--|--|--|--|
| U | | | | | | | |
| BM | | | | | | | |

### TIMES UP DURING THE NIGHT

_____   _____   _____   _____   _____

### TODAY I HAD A SHOWER/WASHED MY HAIR/SPONGE BATH

| Breakfast | |
|-----------|--|
| AM Snack | |
| Lunch | |
| PM Snack | |
| Dinner | |
| Drinks | |

### ACTIVITIES & OTHER COMMENTS

_____

_____

_____

_____

_____

_____

APPOINTMENTS: _____

HEALTH CONCERNS: _____

PLANS FOR TOMORROW: _____

PAIN LEVEL: _____ HAPPINESS LEVEL: _____ ALERTNESS LEVEL: _____

SUPPLIES NEEDED SOON: _____

MEDICATION TAKEN: _____

### NOTES

_____

_____

_____

# Activity & Caregiving Notes for _____ Date: _____

## TOILETING

| TIME | | | | | | | |
|------|--|--|--|--|--|--|--|
| **U** | | | | | | | |
| **BM** | | | | | | | |

### TIMES UP DURING THE NIGHT

_____ _____ _____ _____ _____

### TODAY I HAD A SHOWER/WASHED MY HAIR/SPONGE BATH

| Breakfast | |
|-----------|--|
| AM Snack | |
| Lunch | |
| PM Snack | |
| Dinner | |
| Drinks | |

### ACTIVITIES & OTHER COMMENTS

_____
_____
_____
_____
_____
_____

APPOINTMENTS: _____

HEALTH CONCERNS: _____

PLANS FOR TOMORROW: _____

PAIN LEVEL: _____HAPPINESS LEVEL:_____ALERTNESS LEVEL: _____

SUPPLIES NEEDED SOON:_____

MEDICATION TAKEN:_____

### NOTES

_____
_____
_____

# Activity & Caregiving Notes for _____ Date: _____

## TOILETING

| TIME | | | | | | | |
|------|--|--|--|--|--|--|--|
| U | | | | | | | |
| BM | | | | | | | |

## TIMES UP DURING THE NIGHT

_____   _____   _____   _____   _____

## TODAY I HAD A SHOWER/WASHED MY HAIR/SPONGE BATH

| Breakfast | |
|-----------|--|
| AM Snack | |
| Lunch | |
| PM Snack | |
| Dinner | |
| Drinks | |

## ACTIVITIES & OTHER COMMENTS

_____
_____
_____
_____
_____
_____

APPOINTMENTS: _____

HEALTH CONCERNS: _____

PLANS FOR TOMORROW: _____

PAIN LEVEL: _____ HAPPINESS LEVEL:_____ ALERTNESS LEVEL: _____

SUPPLIES NEEDED SOON: _____

MEDICATION TAKEN: _____

## NOTES

_____
_____
_____

# Activity & Caregiving Notes for _____ Date: _____

## TOILETING

| TIME | | | | | | | |
|------|--|--|--|--|--|--|--|
| U | | | | | | | |
| BM | | | | | | | |

TIMES UP DURING THE NIGHT

_____  _____  _____  _____  _____

TODAY I HAD A SHOWER/WASHED MY HAIR/SPONGE BATH

| Breakfast | |
|-----------|--|
| AM Snack | |
| Lunch | |
| PM Snack | |
| Dinner | |
| Drinks | |

## ACTIVITIES & OTHER COMMENTS

_____

_____

_____

_____

_____

_____

APPOINTMENTS: _____

HEALTH CONCERNS: _____

PLANS FOR TOMORROW: _____

PAIN LEVEL: _____ HAPPINESS LEVEL: _____ ALERTNESS LEVEL: _____

SUPPLIES NEEDED SOON: _____

MEDICATION TAKEN: _____

## NOTES

_____

_____

_____

# Activity & Caregiving Notes for _____ Date: _____

### TOILETING

| TIME | | | | | | |
|------|--|--|--|--|--|--|
| U | | | | | | |
| BM | | | | | | |

### TIMES UP DURING THE NIGHT

_____   _____   _____   _____   _____

### TODAY I HAD A SHOWER/WASHED MY HAIR/SPONGE BATH

| Breakfast | |
|-----------|--|
| AM Snack | |
| Lunch | |
| PM Snack | |
| Dinner | |
| Drinks | |

### ACTIVITIES & OTHER COMMENTS

_____

_____

_____

_____

_____

_____

APPOINTMENTS: _____

HEALTH CONCERNS: _____

PLANS FOR TOMORROW: _____

PAIN LEVEL: _____ HAPPINESS LEVEL: _____ ALERTNESS LEVEL: _____

SUPPLIES NEEDED SOON: _____

MEDICATION TAKEN: _____

### NOTES

_____

_____

_____

# Activity & Caregiving Notes for _____ Date: _____

## TOILETING

| TIME | | | | | | | |
|------|--|--|--|--|--|--|--|
| U | | | | | | | |
| BM | | | | | | | |

### TIMES UP DURING THE NIGHT

_____   _____   _____   _____   _____

### TODAY I HAD A SHOWER/WASHED MY HAIR/SPONGE BATH

| Breakfast | |
|-----------|--|
| AM Snack | |
| Lunch | |
| PM Snack | |
| Dinner | |
| Drinks | |

### ACTIVITIES & OTHER COMMENTS

_____
_____
_____
_____
_____
_____

APPOINTMENTS: _____

HEALTH CONCERNS: _____

PLANS FOR TOMORROW: _____

PAIN LEVEL: _____HAPPINESS LEVEL:_____ALERTNESS LEVEL: _____

SUPPLIES NEEDED SOON:_____

MEDICATION TAKEN:_____

### NOTES

_____
_____
_____

# Activity & Caregiving Notes for _____ Date: _____

## TOILETING

| TIME | | | | | | | |
|------|--|--|--|--|--|--|--|
| U | | | | | | | |
| BM | | | | | | | |

### TIMES UP DURING THE NIGHT

_____  _____  _____  _____  _____

### TODAY I HAD A SHOWER/WASHED MY HAIR/SPONGE BATH

| Breakfast | |
|-----------|--|
| AM Snack | |
| Lunch | |
| PM Snack | |
| Dinner | |
| Drinks | |

### ACTIVITIES & OTHER COMMENTS

_____
_____
_____
_____
_____
_____

APPOINTMENTS: _____

HEALTH CONCERNS: _____

PLANS FOR TOMORROW: _____

PAIN LEVEL: _____ HAPPINESS LEVEL: _____ ALERTNESS LEVEL: _____

SUPPLIES NEEDED SOON: _____

MEDICATION TAKEN: _____

### NOTES

_____
_____
_____

# Activity & Caregiving Notes for _____ Date: _____

## TOILETING

| TIME | | | | | | | | |
|------|--|--|--|--|--|--|--|--|
| U | | | | | | | | |
| BM | | | | | | | | |

### TIMES UP DURING THE NIGHT

_____    _____    _____    _____    _____

### TODAY I HAD A SHOWER/WASHED MY HAIR/SPONGE BATH

| Breakfast | |
|-----------|--|
| AM Snack | |
| Lunch | |
| PM Snack | |
| Dinner | |
| Drinks | |

### ACTIVITIES & OTHER COMMENTS

_____

_____

_____

_____

_____

_____

APPOINTMENTS: _____

HEALTH CONCERNS: _____

PLANS FOR TOMORROW:_____

PAIN LEVEL: _____HAPPINESS LEVEL:_____ALERTNESS LEVEL: _____

SUPPLIES NEEDED SOON:_____

MEDICATION TAKEN:_____

### NOTES

_____

_____

_____

# Activity & Caregiving Notes for _____ Date: _____

### TOILETING

| TIME | | | | | | | |
|------|---|---|---|---|---|---|---|
| U | | | | | | | |
| BM | | | | | | | |

### TIMES UP DURING THE NIGHT

_____    _____    _____    _____    _____

### TODAY I HAD A SHOWER/WASHED MY HAIR/SPONGE BATH

| Breakfast | |
|-----------|---|
| AM Snack | |
| Lunch | |
| PM Snack | |
| Dinner | |
| Drinks | |

### ACTIVITIES & OTHER COMMENTS

_____
_____
_____
_____
_____
_____

APPOINTMENTS: _____

HEALTH CONCERNS: _____

PLANS FOR TOMORROW: _____

PAIN LEVEL: _____ HAPPINESS LEVEL:_____ ALERTNESS LEVEL: _____

SUPPLIES NEEDED SOON: _____

MEDICATION TAKEN:_____

### NOTES

_____
_____
_____

# Activity & Caregiving Notes for _____ Date: _____

## TOILETING

| TIME | | | | | | | |
|------|--|--|--|--|--|--|--|
| U | | | | | | | |
| BM | | | | | | | |

TIMES UP DURING THE NIGHT

_____  _____  _____  _____  _____

TODAY I HAD A SHOWER/WASHED MY HAIR/SPONGE BATH

| Breakfast | |
|-----------|--|
| AM Snack | |
| Lunch | |
| PM Snack | |
| Dinner | |
| Drinks | |

## ACTIVITIES & OTHER COMMENTS

_____
_____
_____
_____
_____
_____

APPOINTMENTS: _____

HEALTH CONCERNS: _____

PLANS FOR TOMORROW: _____

PAIN LEVEL: _____ HAPPINESS LEVEL: _____ ALERTNESS LEVEL: _____

SUPPLIES NEEDED SOON: _____

MEDICATION TAKEN: _____

## NOTES

_____
_____
_____

# Activity & Caregiving Notes for _____ Date: _____

### TOILETING

| TIME | | | | | | | |
|------|---|---|---|---|---|---|---|
| U | | | | | | | |
| BM | | | | | | | |

### TIMES UP DURING THE NIGHT

_____    _____    _____    _____    _____

### TODAY I HAD A SHOWER/WASHED MY HAIR/SPONGE BATH

| Breakfast | |
|-----------|---|
| AM Snack | |
| Lunch | |
| PM Snack | |
| Dinner | |
| Drinks | |

### ACTIVITIES & OTHER COMMENTS

_____

_____

_____

_____

_____

_____

APPOINTMENTS: _____

HEALTH CONCERNS: _____

PLANS FOR TOMORROW: _____

PAIN LEVEL: _____ HAPPINESS LEVEL: _____ ALERTNESS LEVEL: _____

SUPPLIES NEEDED SOON: _____

MEDICATION TAKEN: _____

### NOTES

_____

_____

_____

# Activity & Caregiving Notes for _____ Date: _____

## TOILETING

| TIME | | | | | | | |
|------|--|--|--|--|--|--|--|
| U | | | | | | | |
| BM | | | | | | | |

TIMES UP DURING THE NIGHT

_____    _____    _____    _____    _____

TODAY I HAD A SHOWER/WASHED MY HAIR/SPONGE BATH

| Breakfast | |
|-----------|--|
| AM Snack | |
| Lunch | |
| PM Snack | |
| Dinner | |
| Drinks | |

## ACTIVITIES & OTHER COMMENTS

_____

_____

_____

_____

_____

_____

APPOINTMENTS: _____

HEALTH CONCERNS: _____

PLANS FOR TOMORROW: _____

PAIN LEVEL: _____ HAPPINESS LEVEL: _____ ALERTNESS LEVEL: _____

SUPPLIES NEEDED SOON: _____

MEDICATION TAKEN: _____

## NOTES

_____

_____

_____

# Activity & Caregiving Notes for _____ Date: _____

## TOILETING

| TIME | | | | | | | |
|------|--|--|--|--|--|--|--|
| U | | | | | | | |
| BM | | | | | | | |

## TIMES UP DURING THE NIGHT

_____   _____   _____   _____   _____

## TODAY I HAD A SHOWER/WASHED MY HAIR/SPONGE BATH

| Breakfast | |
|-----------|--|
| AM Snack | |
| Lunch | |
| PM Snack | |
| Dinner | |
| Drinks | |

## ACTIVITIES & OTHER COMMENTS

_____

_____

_____

_____

_____

_____

APPOINTMENTS: _____

HEALTH CONCERNS: _____

PLANS FOR TOMORROW: _____

PAIN LEVEL: _____ HAPPINESS LEVEL:_____ALERTNESS LEVEL: _____

SUPPLIES NEEDED SOON:_____

MEDICATION TAKEN:_____

## NOTES

_____

_____

_____

# Activity & Caregiving Notes for _____ Date: _____

### TOILETING

| TIME | | | | | | | |
|------|--|--|--|--|--|--|--|
| U | | | | | | | |
| BM | | | | | | | |

### TIMES UP DURING THE NIGHT

_____  _____  _____  _____  _____

### TODAY I HAD A SHOWER/WASHED MY HAIR/SPONGE BATH

| Breakfast | |
|-----------|--|
| AM Snack | |
| Lunch | |
| PM Snack | |
| Dinner | |
| Drinks | |

### ACTIVITIES & OTHER COMMENTS

_____

_____

_____

_____

_____

_____

APPOINTMENTS: _____

HEALTH CONCERNS: _____

PLANS FOR TOMORROW:_____

PAIN LEVEL: _____HAPPINESS LEVEL:_____ALERTNESS LEVEL: _____

SUPPLIES NEEDED SOON:_____

MEDICATION TAKEN:_____

### NOTES

_____

_____

_____

# Activity & Caregiving Notes for _____ Date: _____

### TOILETING

| TIME | | | | | | | |
|------|--|--|--|--|--|--|--|
| U | | | | | | | |
| BM | | | | | | | |

### TIMES UP DURING THE NIGHT

_____  _____  _____  _____  _____

### TODAY I HAD A SHOWER/WASHED MY HAIR/SPONGE BATH

| Breakfast | |
|-----------|--|
| AM Snack | |
| Lunch | |
| PM Snack | |
| Dinner | |
| Drinks | |

### ACTIVITIES & OTHER COMMENTS

_____
_____
_____
_____
_____
_____

APPOINTMENTS: _____
HEALTH CONCERNS: _____
PLANS FOR TOMORROW: _____
PAIN LEVEL: _____HAPPINESS LEVEL:_____ALERTNESS LEVEL: _____
SUPPLIES NEEDED SOON: _____
MEDICATION TAKEN: _____

### NOTES

_____
_____
_____

# Activity & Caregiving Notes for _____ Date: _____

## TOILETING

| TIME | | | | | | | |
|------|--|--|--|--|--|--|--|
| U | | | | | | | |
| BM | | | | | | | |

TIMES UP DURING THE NIGHT

_____ _____ _____ _____ _____

TODAY I HAD A SHOWER/WASHED MY HAIR/SPONGE BATH

| Breakfast | |
|-----------|--|
| AM Snack | |
| Lunch | |
| PM Snack | |
| Dinner | |
| Drinks | |

## ACTIVITIES & OTHER COMMENTS

_____

_____

_____

_____

_____

_____

APPOINTMENTS: _____

HEALTH CONCERNS: _____

PLANS FOR TOMORROW: _____

PAIN LEVEL: _____ HAPPINESS LEVEL: _____ ALERTNESS LEVEL: _____

SUPPLIES NEEDED SOON: _____

MEDICATION TAKEN: _____

## NOTES

_____

_____

_____

# Activity & Caregiving Notes for _____ Date: _____

## TOILETING

| TIME | | | | | | | |
|------|---|---|---|---|---|---|---|
| U | | | | | | | |
| BM | | | | | | | |

TIMES UP DURING THE NIGHT

_____  _____  _____  _____  _____

TODAY I HAD A SHOWER/WASHED MY HAIR/SPONGE BATH

| Breakfast | |
|-----------|---|
| AM Snack | |
| Lunch | |
| PM Snack | |
| Dinner | |
| Drinks | |

## ACTIVITIES & OTHER COMMENTS

_____

_____

_____

_____

_____

_____

APPOINTMENTS: _____

HEALTH CONCERNS: _____

PLANS FOR TOMORROW: _____

PAIN LEVEL: _____ HAPPINESS LEVEL: _____ ALERTNESS LEVEL: _____

SUPPLIES NEEDED SOON: _____

MEDICATION TAKEN: _____

## NOTES

_____

_____

_____

# Activity & Caregiving Notes for _____ Date: _____

TOILETING

| TIME | | | | | | | |
|------|--|--|--|--|--|--|--|
| U | | | | | | | |
| BM | | | | | | | |

TIMES UP DURING THE NIGHT

_____   _____   _____   _____   _____

TODAY I HAD A SHOWER/WASHED MY HAIR/SPONGE BATH

| Breakfast | |
|-----------|--|
| AM Snack | |
| Lunch | |
| PM Snack | |
| Dinner | |
| Drinks | |

ACTIVITIES & OTHER COMMENTS

_____

_____

_____

_____

_____

_____

APPOINTMENTS: _____

HEALTH CONCERNS: _____

PLANS FOR TOMORROW: _____

PAIN LEVEL: _____ HAPPINESS LEVEL: _____ ALERTNESS LEVEL: _____

SUPPLIES NEEDED SOON: _____

MEDICATION TAKEN: _____

NOTES

_____

_____

_____

# Activity & Caregiving Notes for _____ Date: _____

## TOILETING

| TIME | | | | | | | |
|------|--|--|--|--|--|--|--|
| U | | | | | | | |
| BM | | | | | | | |

### TIMES UP DURING THE NIGHT

_____    _____    _____    _____    _____

### TODAY I HAD A SHOWER/WASHED MY HAIR/SPONGE BATH

| Breakfast | |
|-----------|--|
| AM Snack | |
| Lunch | |
| PM Snack | |
| Dinner | |
| Drinks | |

### ACTIVITIES & OTHER COMMENTS

_____
_____
_____
_____
_____
_____

APPOINTMENTS: _____

HEALTH CONCERNS: _____

PLANS FOR TOMORROW:_____

PAIN LEVEL: _____HAPPINESS LEVEL:_____ALERTNESS LEVEL: _____

SUPPLIES NEEDED SOON:_____

MEDICATION TAKEN:_____

### NOTES

_____
_____
_____

# Activity & Caregiving Notes for _____ Date: _____

## TOILETING

| TIME | | | | | | | |
|------|---|---|---|---|---|---|---|
| U | | | | | | | |
| BM | | | | | | | |

### TIMES UP DURING THE NIGHT

_____    _____    _____    _____    _____

### TODAY I HAD A SHOWER/WASHED MY HAIR/SPONGE BATH

| Breakfast | |
|-----------|---|
| AM Snack | |
| Lunch | |
| PM Snack | |
| Dinner | |
| Drinks | |

### ACTIVITIES & OTHER COMMENTS

_____

_____

_____

_____

_____

_____

APPOINTMENTS: _____

HEALTH CONCERNS: _____

PLANS FOR TOMORROW: _____

PAIN LEVEL: _____HAPPINESS LEVEL:_____ALERTNESS LEVEL: _____

SUPPLIES NEEDED SOON:_____

MEDICATION TAKEN:_____

### NOTES

_____

_____

_____

# Activity & Caregiving Notes for _____ Date: _____

### TOILETING

| TIME | | | | | | | |
|------|---|---|---|---|---|---|---|
| U | | | | | | | |
| BM | | | | | | | |

### TIMES UP DURING THE NIGHT

_____ _____ _____ _____ _____

### TODAY I HAD A SHOWER/WASHED MY HAIR/SPONGE BATH

| Breakfast | |
|-----------|---|
| AM Snack | |
| Lunch | |
| PM Snack | |
| Dinner | |
| Drinks | |

### ACTIVITIES & OTHER COMMENTS

_____

_____

_____

_____

_____

_____

APPOINTMENTS: _____

HEALTH CONCERNS: _____

PLANS FOR TOMORROW: _____

PAIN LEVEL: _____ HAPPINESS LEVEL: _____ ALERTNESS LEVEL: _____

SUPPLIES NEEDED SOON: _____

MEDICATION TAKEN: _____

### NOTES

_____

_____

_____

# Activity & Caregiving Notes for _____ Date: _____

## TOILETING

| TIME | | | | | | | |
|------|--|--|--|--|--|--|--|
| U | | | | | | | |
| BM | | | | | | | |

### TIMES UP DURING THE NIGHT

_____  _____  _____  _____  _____

### TODAY I HAD A SHOWER/WASHED MY HAIR/SPONGE BATH

| Breakfast | |
|-----------|--|
| AM Snack | |
| Lunch | |
| PM Snack | |
| Dinner | |
| Drinks | |

### ACTIVITIES & OTHER COMMENTS

_____

_____

_____

_____

_____

_____

APPOINTMENTS: _____

HEALTH CONCERNS: _____

PLANS FOR TOMORROW: _____

PAIN LEVEL: _____HAPPINESS LEVEL:_____ALERTNESS LEVEL: _____

SUPPLIES NEEDED SOON:_____

MEDICATION TAKEN:_____

### NOTES

_____

_____

_____